CONTENTS

01. KETO BREAD LOAVES

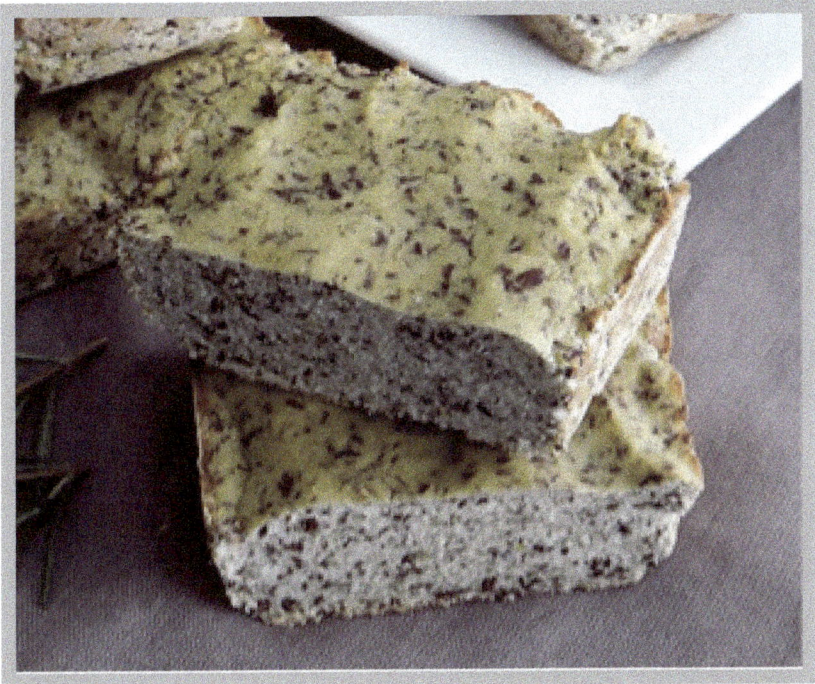

*P*reparation time: 15 min
Cooking time: 40 min

Ready in: 55 min

Ingredients:

1. 6 large eggs

2. 1 cup coconut flour, sifted

3. ½ cup flaxseed meal

4. 1 teaspoon salt

5. 1 teaspoon baking powder

6. ½ teaspoon baking soda

7. ½ cup water

8. 1 tablespoon apple cider vinegar

Instructions:

1. At first, preheat your oven to 350F and grease pan(s) and then sift the coconut flour into a mixing bowl.

2. Then add remaining dry ingredients and whisk.

3. Plus, eggs, water, and vinegar.

4. Then stir until batter comes together. It will be thick.

5. Please press the batter into pan(s) and bake until cooked through about 40 minutes.

6. At the final stage, please allow the bread to cool in pan until just warm, then remove from pan, slice, and enjoy.

02. SUPER EASY KETO BREAD

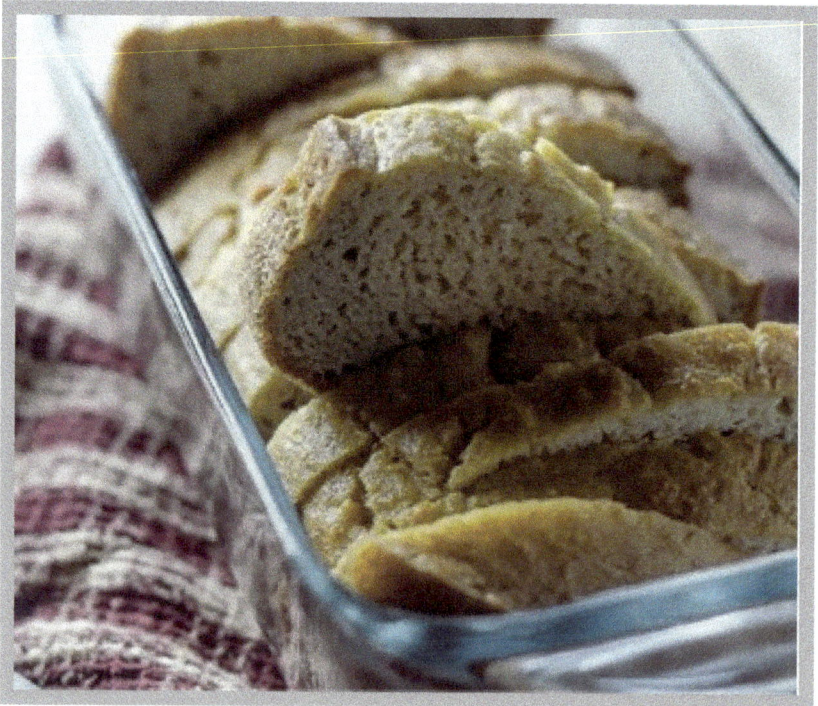

*P*reparation time: 5 min

Cooking time: 30 min

Ready in: 35 min

Ingredients:

1. 1-1/4 cup blanched almond flour (150 g)

2. 1/3 cup coconut flour (37 g)

3. 1 teaspoon baking soda

4. 3 tablespoons coconut oil or butter melted

5. 2 teaspoons apple cider vinegar

6. 8 large eggs

Instructions:

1. Do preheat oven 350F.

2. Then grease a bread pan with coconut oil or butter, making sure to coat the entire interior of the pan.

3. Now mix dry ingredients together in a bowl. Please mix wet ingredients together in another bowl.

4. Then add half of the wet ingredients to the dry ingredients and mix well and add remaining wet ingredients and mix again. Now pour the mixture into a greased dish and place in oven. Please bake for 30-35 minutes, or until the edges have browned.

5. Now remove from oven and allow cooling to the touch before removing from pan and slicing. Then serve immediately, or allow cooling to room temperature before storing in an air-tight container. It can be stored at room temperature for 3-4 days. If you want, then you can store in the fridge for up to a week or in the freezer for up to a month.

6. Last stage: Slice before freezing and thaw in the microwave or at room temperature.

03. KETO/LOW CARB LOAF BREAD

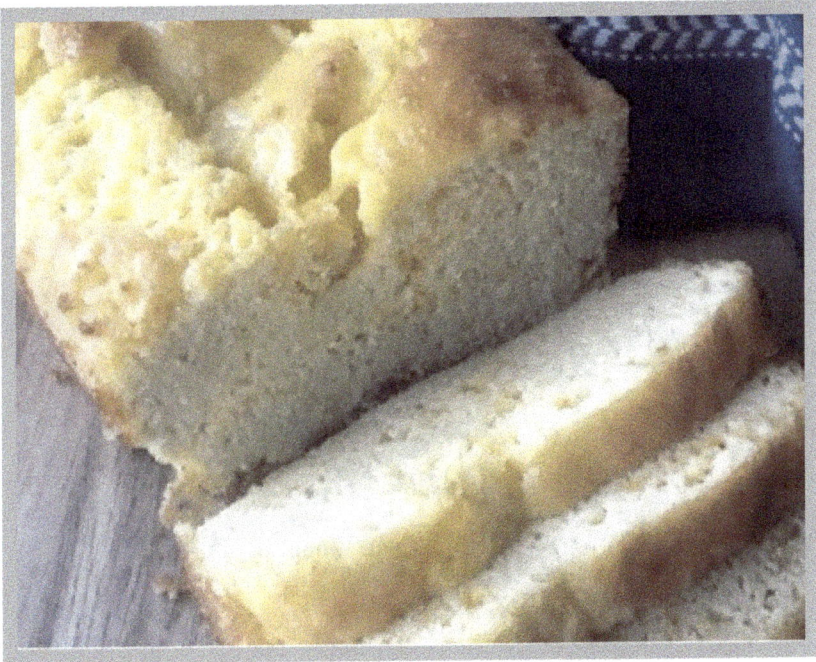

*P*reparation time: 10 min

Cooking time: 45 min

Ready in: 55 min

Ingredients:

1. 1/2 cup coconut flour
2. 10 tbsp butter, melted
3. 8 eggs
4. 2 tbsp sour cream
5. 1 1/2 tsp baking powder
6. 1/2 cup cheddar cheese

Instructions:

1. Do preheat oven to 350.
2. Now melt butter and set aside until it is room temperature.
3. Please add all other ingredients and stir to combine.
4. Then grease loaf pan or line with parchment paper.
5. Please pour the batter in a loaf pan and cook for 45-50 minutes or until a toothpick inserted in the center of the loaf comes out clean.
6. Final stage: Before serving, fry each slice in butter in a skillet or toast in the air fryer or toaster oven. Remind this step is key to a piece of great tasting bread.

04. THE BEST KETO BREAD RECIPE

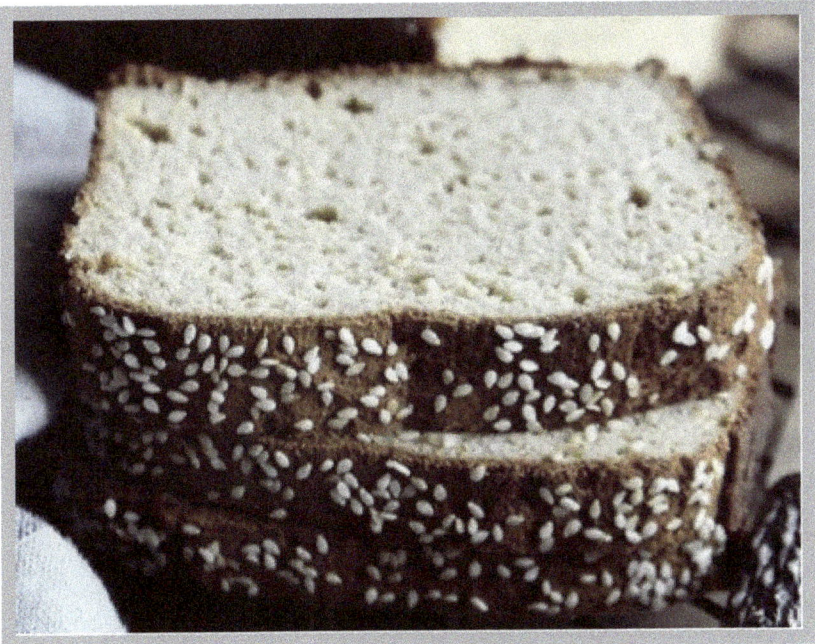

$\mathcal{P}$ reparation time: 15 min

Cooking time: 90 min

Ready in: 105 min

Ingredients:

1. Avocado oil

2. 2 cups almond flour

3. 3/4 cup coconut flour

4. 2 tablespoons husk powder

5. 1 teaspoon salt

6. 2 teaspoons baking powder

7. 2 teaspoons instant yeast

8. 2 tablespoons warm water

9. 2 teaspoons coconut sugar

10. 1 tablespoon grass-fed beef gelatin

11. 3 tablespoons boiling water

12. 1 cup egg whites at room temperature

13. 2 tablespoons apple cider vinegar

14. 5 drops liquid stevia

15. 6 tablespoons grass-fed clarified butter ghee, melted and cooled slightly

16. 3/4 cup boiling water

17. 1 teaspoon sesame seeds

Instructions:

1. At first, preheat oven to 350F; line the inside of a 9 by 5-inch loaf pan with parchment paper and lightly spray the inside with avocado oil.

2. Then whisk together the almond flour, coconut flour, husk powder, salt, and baking powder in a large bowl.

3. Please stir together the yeast, 2 tablespoons warm water, and coconut sugar in a small bowl and let it sit 12 minutes until foamy.

4. Now stir together the gelatin and 3 tablespoons boiling water in a small bowl until fully dissolved.

5. Then stir together the dissolved yeast, dissolved beef gelatin, egg whites, vinegar, liquid stevia, and melted ghee in a medium bowl.

6. And then stir the egg white mixture into the dry ingredients, and then beat in the 3/4 cup boiling water.

7. Do immediately pour the dough into the prepared loaf pan and smooth out the top and let it rest for 4 minutes. Now sprinkle the sesame seeds on top.

8. Please bake until a wooden pick inserted in the center comes out clean, about 1 hour 14 minutes to 1 hour 33 minutes, for covering the top with foil to prevent over-browning if necessary. Now the loaf is done when it sounds hollow when tapped on the bottom.

9. Please turn off the oven, leave the door ajar, and let the bread cool for 30 minutes in the warm oven.

10. at this stage, transfer the bread to a wire rack to finish cooling before slicing.

05. KETO GARLIC BREAD

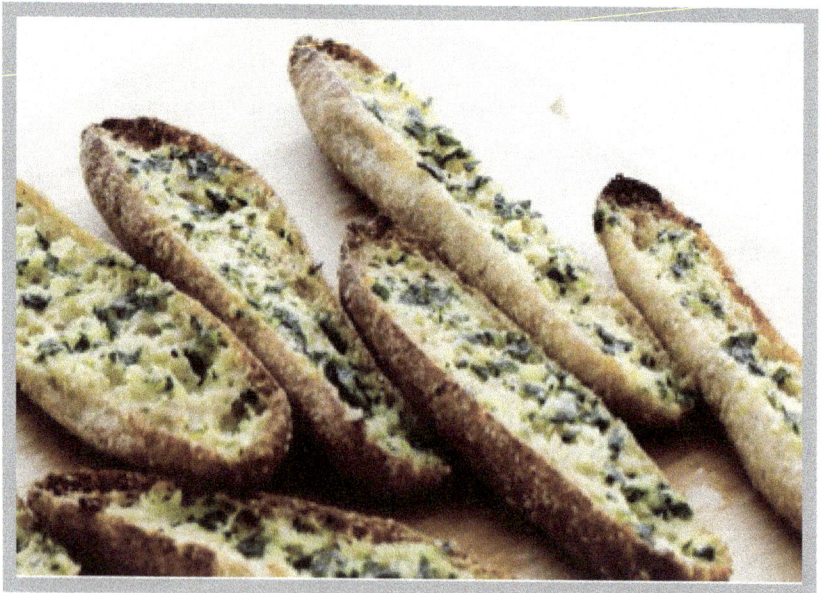

*P*reparation time: 10 min

Cooking time: 65 min

Ready in: 75 min

. . .

Ingredients:

Bread:

1. 1¼ cups almond flour

2. 5 tbsp ground husk powder

3. 2 tsp baking powder

4. 1 tsp sea salt

5. 2 tsp cider vinegar or white wine vinegar

6. 1 cup boiling water

7. 3 egg whites

Garlic butter:

1. 4 oz. butter, at room temperature

2. 1 garlic clove, minced

3. 2 tbsp fresh parsley, finely chopped

4. ½ tsp salt

Instructions:

1. On preheat the oven to 350°F (175°C) and mix the dry ingredients for the bread in a bowl.

2. Following the first step please bring the water to a boil and add this, the vinegar and egg whites to the bowl, while whisking with a hand mixer for about 31 seconds. Please don't over mix the dough; the consistency should resemble Play-Doh.

3. Now form with moist hands into 10 pieces and roll into hot dog buns. Please make sure to leave enough space between them on the baking sheet to double in size.

4. Do bake on lower rack in oven for 45-50 minutes; they're done when you can hear a hollow sound when tapping the bottom of the bun.

5. Please make the garlic butter while the bread is baking and mix all the ingredients together and put it in the fridge.

6. Please take the buns out of the oven when they're done and leave to let cool and take the garlic butter out of the fridge. Notice one thing when the buns are cooled, cut them in halves, using a serrated knife, and spread garlic butter on each half.

7. Please turn your oven up to 425°F (225°C) and bake the garlic bread for 11-15 minutes, until golden brown.

06. FLUFFY KETO BREAD RECIPE

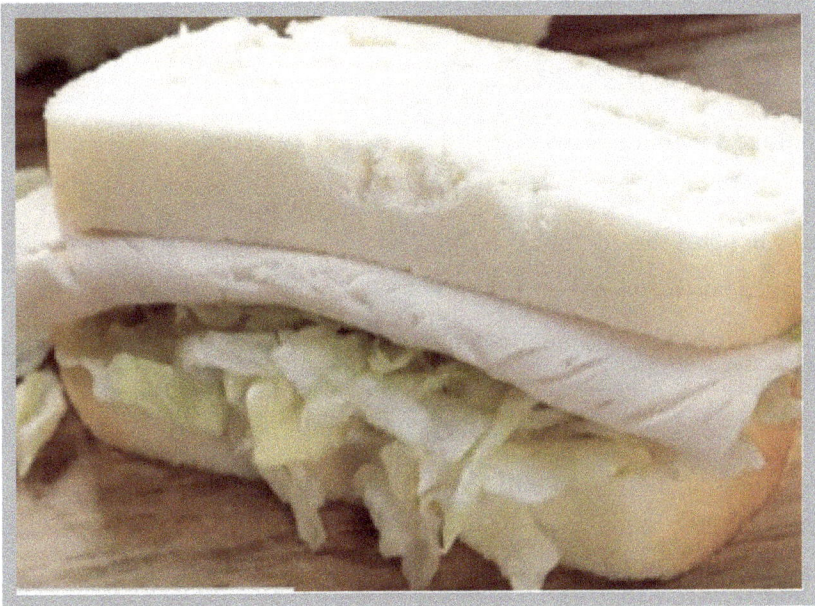

*P*reparation time: 10 min

Cooking time: 30 min

Ready in: 40 min

Ingredients:

1. 8 large egg whites or 1 cup of egg whites

2. 1/2 cup cream cheese

3. 1 tsp baking powder

4. 2 tbs sparkling mineral water

5. 1 cup almond flour

Instructions:

1. Take a medium bowl, add the egg whites. Now use a hand mixer to mix them until they have doubled in size and are soft and frothy.

2. Then add the cream cheese and continue using the hand mixer on high speed until it's fully mixed and smooth in texture.

3. Now add the baking powder, sparkling mineral water, and almond flour. Please use the hand mixer on medium speed until it's fully combined.

4. Now pour the mixture in a greased 9 x 5 bread loaf pan.

5. Do bake it at 350 degrees for about 25 minutes or until the center is fully cooked and its golden brown on top. If you want, then you can poke a toothpick in the center of the bread and if the toothpick comes out clean,

6. it's done.

07. THE BEST LOW CARB BREAD RECIPE {NO EGG TASTE}

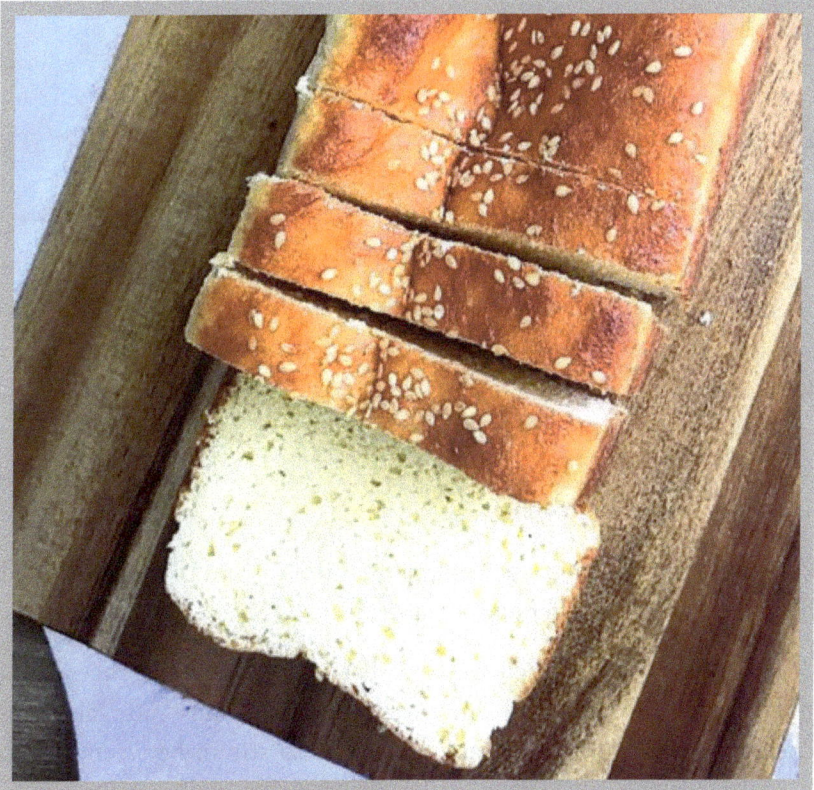

$\mathcal{P}$ reparation time: 8 min

Cooking time: 15 min

Ready in: 23 min

Ingredients:

1. 1 1/2 cup almond flour

2. 1 tbsp Baking powder

3. 2 1/2 cup shredded Mozzarella cheese

4. 2 Tbsp Cream cheese

5. 2 large Egg

6. 7 g active dry or instant dry yeast

7. Sesame seeds (optional)

8. 1 tbsp erythritol (optional)

Instructions:

1. On preheat oven to 400ºF

2. Then mix dry ingredients (almond flour, yeast, erythritol, and baking powder) together and set aside

3. Please put the cream cheese and shredded Mozzarella cheese in a microwave-safe bowl and microwave in 28 seconds intervals until cheese is evenly melted. Please remember to stir in between (which

helps to distribute the heat.) it usually takes me about 1 min 30 secs in total sometimes 2.30 mins.

4. Now pour dry ingredients into the microwaved cheese mix the and mix with your hands or with a spatula then add the cold eggs and mix till a ball of dough forms

5. Now transfer to a loaf pan lined with parchment

6. Then sprinkle sesame seeds on top if using and then bake in the oven for 12 to 15 mins or until the top is golden brown

7. Last part: Bring out of the oven, allow cooling, and enjoying.

08. KETO BREAD WITH ALMOND FLOUR

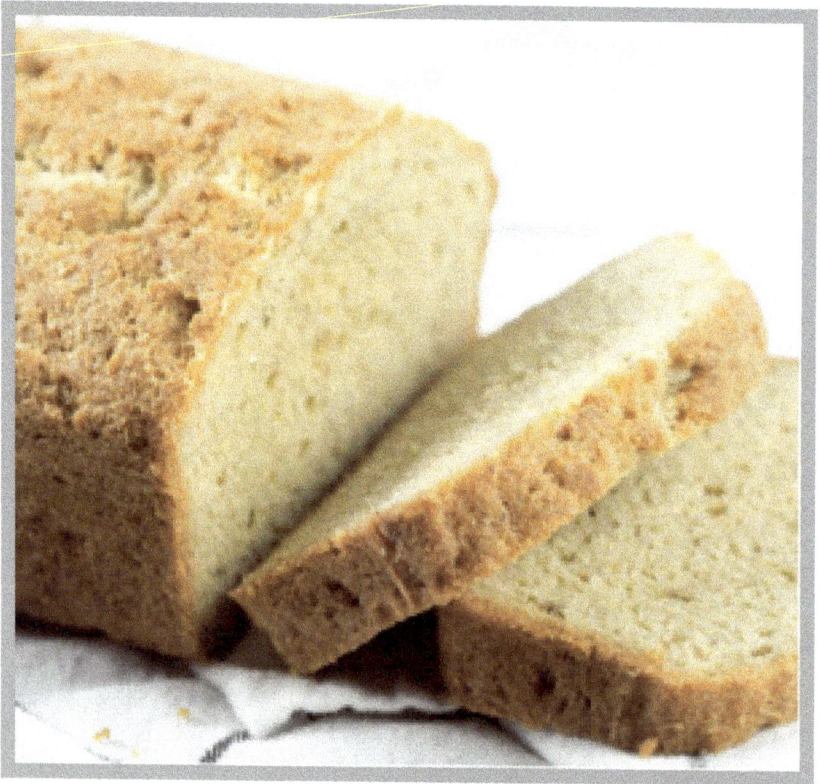

*P*reparation time: 15 min

Cooking time: 30 min

Ready in: 45 min

Ingredients:

1. 1 1/2 cups almond flour

2. 1/4 cup husk fiber

3. 2 Tablespoons baking powder

4. 6 whole eggs

5. 3/4 cup coconut oil, melted

6. 1/4 teaspoon salt

Instructions:

1. At first, preheat oven to 375 degrees F and line a standard bread loaf pan with parchment paper.

2. Then in a medium mixing bowl, whisk together all of the ingredients until well combined.

3. now pour the batter into the loaf pan and "tap/drop the pan" from about a 1/2 inch height onto your countertop a few times to work the air bubbles out of the batter.

4. Please bake for 30 minutes or until a knife inserted into the middle of the loaf pulls out clean.

5. At last, please allow the bread to cool in pan before removing and slicing fully.

09. MY FAVORITE KETO BREAD

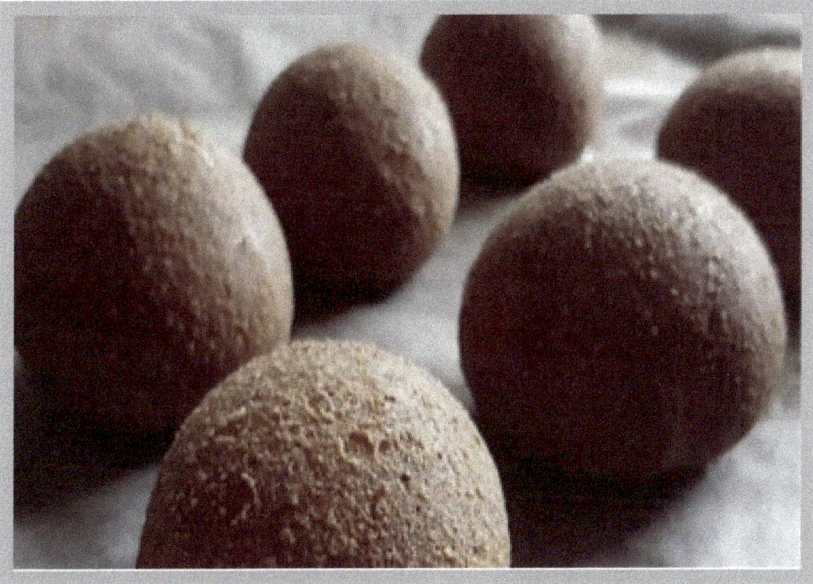

*P*reparation time: 10 min

Cooking time: 55 min

Ready in: 65 min

. . .

Ingredients:

1. 1½ cups blanched almond flour

2. 5 tablespoons husk powder

3. 2 teaspoons baking powder

4. 1 teaspoon Celtic sea salt

5. 2½ tablespoons apple cider vinegar

6. 3 egg whites (6 if using coconut flour)

7. 7/8 cup (a little less than a cup) boiling water

Instructions:

1. At first, preheat the oven to 350°F.

2. Take a medium-sized bowl, combine the flour, powder (no substitutes: flaxseed meal won't work), baking powder and salt, and mix until dry ingredients are well combined.

3. Then add in the eggs and vinegar and mix until a thick dough and add boiling water or marinara into the bowl. Now mix until well combined and dough firms up.

4. Now form into 4 to 5 mini subs (the dough will rise about 2 to 3

times, so I start mine as a 1-inch disk) or one large sub/loaf and place onto a greased baking sheet.

5. Please bake for 50 minutes (45-50 minutes for smaller shapes like buns) and remove from the oven and allow the bread to cool completely.

6. Now cut open with a serrated knife and fill with desired keto-friendly toppings.

10. BEST KETO BREAD – LOW CARB, PALEO

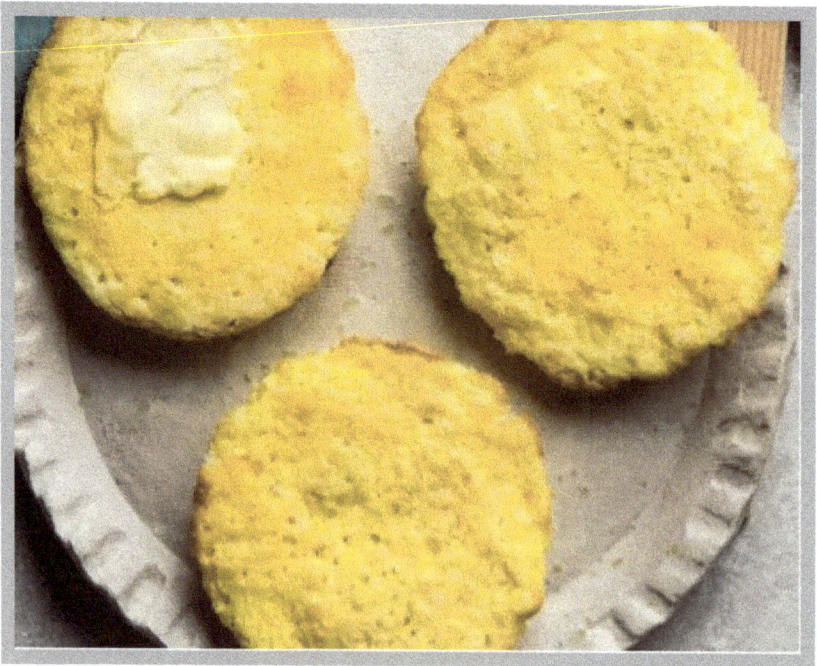

*P*reparation time: 5 min

Cooking time: 10 min

Ready in: 15 min

Ingredients:

1. 1 1/2 tablespoons ghee, (softened)

2. In alternative 1 1/2 tablespoons buttery flavored coconut oil, (softened)

3. 1 large egg

4. 1/2 teaspoon baking powder

5. Pinch garlic powder

6. 1 1/2 tablespoon coconut flour OR 1/4 cup super-fine almond flour (only one)

7. Pinch pink salt, optional

Instructions:

1. at first coat, a 12-ounce mug or ramekin with coconut oil or ghee for easier removal. Then add the ghee and egg and whisk together with a fork until smooth and add the baking powder, garlic powder, optional salt, and coconut flour and stir until combined.

To cook in the microwave:

. . .

1. Please place it in a microwave and cook on HIGH for 90 seconds.

To cook in the oven:

1. Do bake in a preheated oven at 400F for 8-10 minutes.

11. KETO BREAD 1

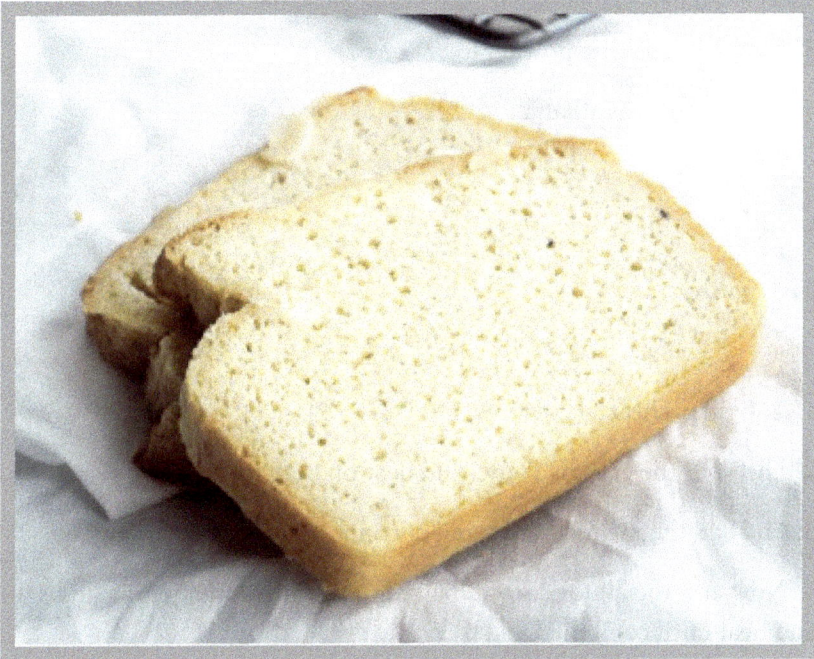

*P*reparation time: 15 min

Cooking time: 40 min

Ready in: 55 min

Ingredients:

1. 7 Large Eggs (50g / 1.7 oz each)

2. 3.5 oz Butter melted (100 g / 1/2 cup)

3. 1 oz Coconut Oil (30 g / 2 Tbsp)

4. 7 oz Almond Flour (200 g / 2 Cups)

5. 1 teaspoon baking powder (5g / 0.2 oz)

6. 1/2 teaspoon xanthan gum (2g)

7. 1/2 teaspoon salt (2g)

Instructions:

1. At first, preheat the oven to 180 C (355 F).

2. Then put the eggs in a bowl and beat on high for 1 to 2 minutes.

3. And add the melted butter and coconut oil beat until smooth.

4. Now add the almond flour, baking powder, xanthan gum, and salt, and beat until combined and thick.

.   .   .

5. Then scrape into an 8-inch X 4-inch (20 cm x 10 cm) loaf pan lined with baking paper.

6. Do bake for 45 minutes or until a skewer comes out of the middle clean.

7. Do slice into 16 thin slices and store in an airtight container in the fridge for up to 7 days or up to 1 month in the freezer.

12. BEST KETO BREAD

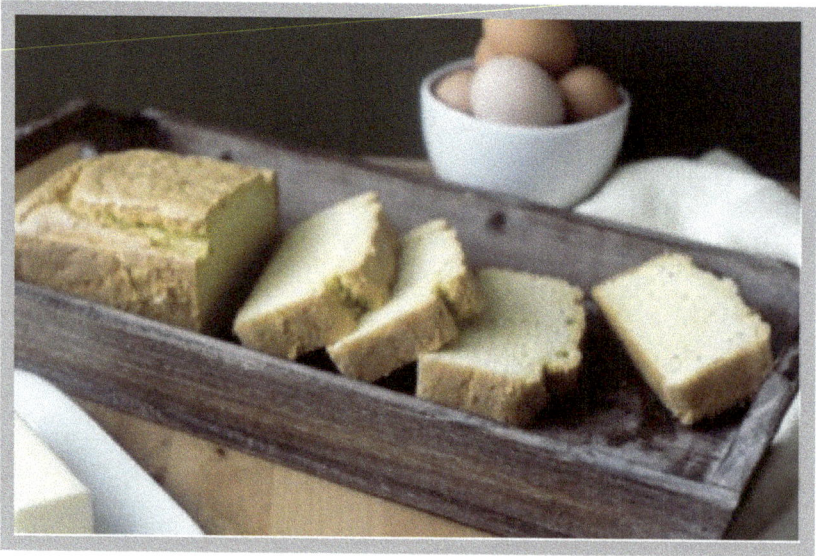

*P*reparation time: 10 min

Cooking time: 30 min

Ready in: 40 min

Ingredients:

1. 1 1/2 Cup Almond Flour

2. 6 large eggs Separated

3. 1/4 cup butter melted

4. 3 tsp Baking powder

5. 1/4 tsp Cream

6. 1 pinch Pink Salt

7. 6 drops Liquid Stevia optional

Instructions:

1. At first, preheat oven to 375.

2. Please separate the egg whites from the yolks and add Cream to the whites and beat until soft peaks are achieved.

3. now in a food processor combine the egg yolks, 1/3 of the beaten egg whites, melted butter, almond flour, baking powder, and salt (Adding 6 drops of liquid stevia to the batter can help reduce the mild egg taste) and mix until combined. When this will be lumpy, thick dough until the whites are added.

4. Then add the remaining 2/3 of the egg whites and gently process until fully incorporated. Please be careful not to over mix as this is what gives the bread it's volume!

5. Now pour the mixture into a buttered 8x4 loaf pan. Do bake for 30 minutes. Please check with a toothpick to ensure the bread is cooked through.

6. Enjoy! 1 loaf makes 20 slices.

13. BEST KETO BREAD 2

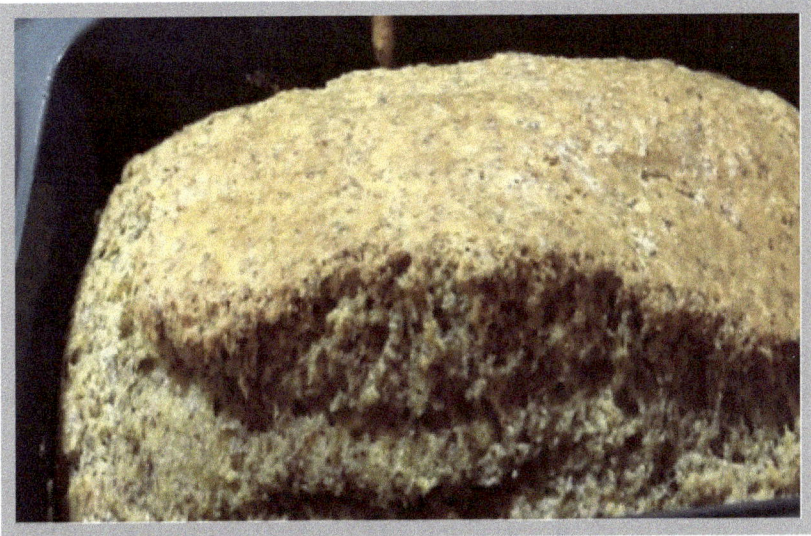

*P*reparation time: 20 min

Cooking time: 40 min

Ready in: 60 min

Ingredients:

1. Cooking spray

2. 7 eggs

3. ½ cup butter melted and cooled

4. 2 tablespoons olive oil

5. 2 cups blanched almond flour

6. 1 teaspoon baking powder

7. ½ teaspoon xanthan gum

8 ½ teaspoon of sea salts

Instructions:

1. First, heat in advance the oven to 350 degrees F (175 degrees C) and grease a silicone loaf pan with cooking spray.

2. Then whisk eggs in a bowl until smooth and creamy, about 3.30 minutes. And add melted butter and olive oil; mix until well combined.

3. Now combine almond flour, baking powder, xanthan gum, and salt in a separate bowl; mix well and add gradually to the egg mixture, mixing well until a thick batter is formed.

4. Following this step please pour batter into the prepared pan and smooth the top with a spatula.

5. Do bake in the preheated oven until a toothpick inserted into the center comes out clean, about 45 minutes.

14. EASY PALEO KETO BREAD RECIPE - 5 INGREDIENTS

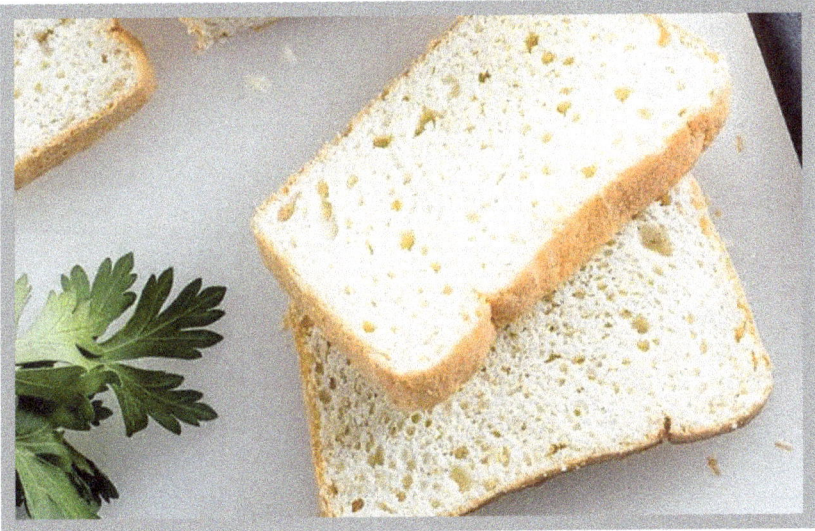

*P*reparation time: 10 min

Cooking time: 70 min

Ready in: 80 min

Ingredients:

Basic Ingredients:

1. 1 cup Blanched almond flour

2. 1/4 cup Coconut flour

3. 2 tsp Gluten-free baking powder

4. 1/4 tsp Sea salt

5. 1/3 cup Butter

6. 12 large Egg white (1 1/2 cups)

Optional Ingredients (recommended):

1. 1 1/2 tbsp Erythritol

2. 1/4 tsp Xanthan gum

3. 1/4 tsp Cream of tartar

Instructions:

1. At first, preheat the oven to 325 degrees F (163 degrees C) and line an 8 1/2 x 4 1/2 in (22x11 cm) loaf pan with parchment paper and with extra hanging over the sides for normal removal later.

2. Then combine the almond flour, coconut flour, baking powder, erythritol, xanthan gum, and sea salt in a large food processor. Please pulse until combined.

3. Then add the melted butter and pulse, scraping down the sides as needed, until crumbly.

4. Now in a very large bowl, use a hand mixer to beat the egg whites and cream of tartar (if using) until stiff peaks form. Please make sure the bowl is large enough because the whites will expand a lot.

5. Then add 1/2 of the stiff egg whites to the food processor and pulse a few times until just combined. Be careful, do not over-mix!

6. Now carefully transfer the mixture from the food processor into the bowl with the egg whites and gently fold until no streaks remain. Remind one thing do not stir. Then fold gently to keep the mixture as fluffy as possible.

7. Then transfer the batter to the lined loaf pan and smooth the top. Please push the batter toward the center a bit to round the top.

8. Do bake for about 38 minutes, until the top is golden brown and tent the top with aluminum foil and bake for another 30-45 minutes, the internal temperature should be 200 degrees. Let's cool completely before removing from the pan and slicing.

15. KETO BREAD 2

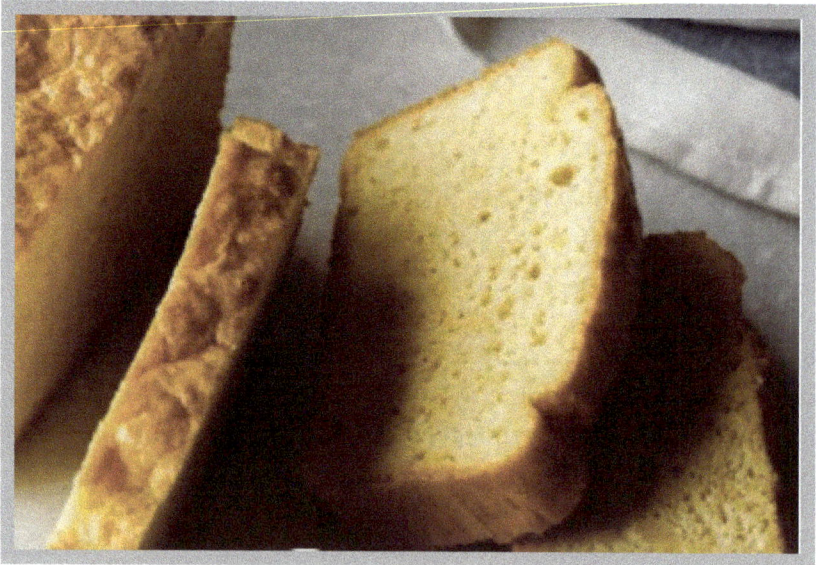

*P*reparation time: 40 min

Cooking time: 80 min

Ready in: 120 min

Ingredients:

1. 1 stick (8 tablespoons)

2. 1 3/4 cups blanched almond flour

3. 2 teaspoons baking powder

4. 1/2 teaspoon kosher salt

5. 6 large eggs,

Instructions:

1. at first preheat the oven to 350 degrees F and butter a 9-by-5-inch loaf pan and line the pan with a piece of parchment paper long enough to have a 2-inch overhang on 2 sides (this will help you lift the bread out of the pan).

2. Then whisk the almond flour, baking powder, and salt together in a large bowl and whisk in the egg yolks and butter.

3. Now beat the egg whites in another large bowl with an electric mixer on medium-high speed until they hold soft peaks and stir about a third of the whipped egg whites into the almond flour mixture. And then gently fold in the remaining egg whites, being careful not to over mix (its okay if there are some egg white streaks in the batter).

4. Please pour the batter into the prepared pan and bake until golden brown and a toothpick inserted in the center comes out clean, 24 to 30 minutes. Now let's cool completely in the pan on a rack. Then use

the parchment to help lift the bread out and slice for sandwiches or toast or eat with a slather of butter.

5. Final stage: Wrap and store at room temperature for up to 5 days.

16. KETO BREAD 3

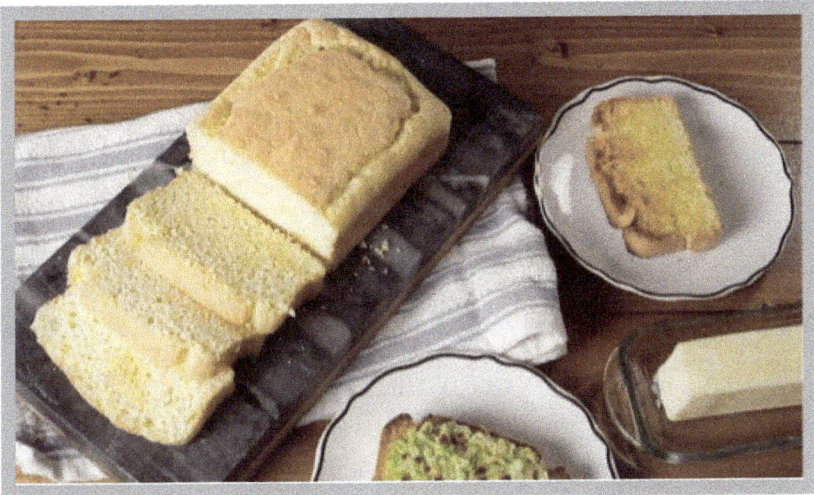

*P*reparation time: 10 min

Cooking time: 60 min

Ready in: 70 min

. . .

Ingredients:

1. 6 large eggs

2. 1/2 tsp. cream of tartar

3. 1/4 c. (1/2 stick) butter, melted and cooled

4. 1 1/2 c. finely ground almond flour

5. 1 tbsp baking powder

6. 1/2 tsp. kosher salt

Instructions:

1. At first, preheat oven to 375° and line an 8"-x-4" loaf pan with parchment paper and separate egg whites and egg yolks.

2. Take a large bowl, combine egg whites and cream of tartar. You have to Use a hand mixer, whip until stiff peaks form.

3. Following this step please prepare in a separate large bowl using a hand mixer, beat yolks with melted butter, almond flour, baking powder, and salt. Now kindly fold in 1/3 of the whipped egg whites until fully incorporated, and then fold in the rest.

4. Please pour batter into loaf pan and smooth top. Bake for 29 minutes, or until the top is slightly golden and a toothpick inserted comes out clean.

5. Lets cool 35 minutes before slicing.

17. 90 SECOND LOW CARB KETO BREAD

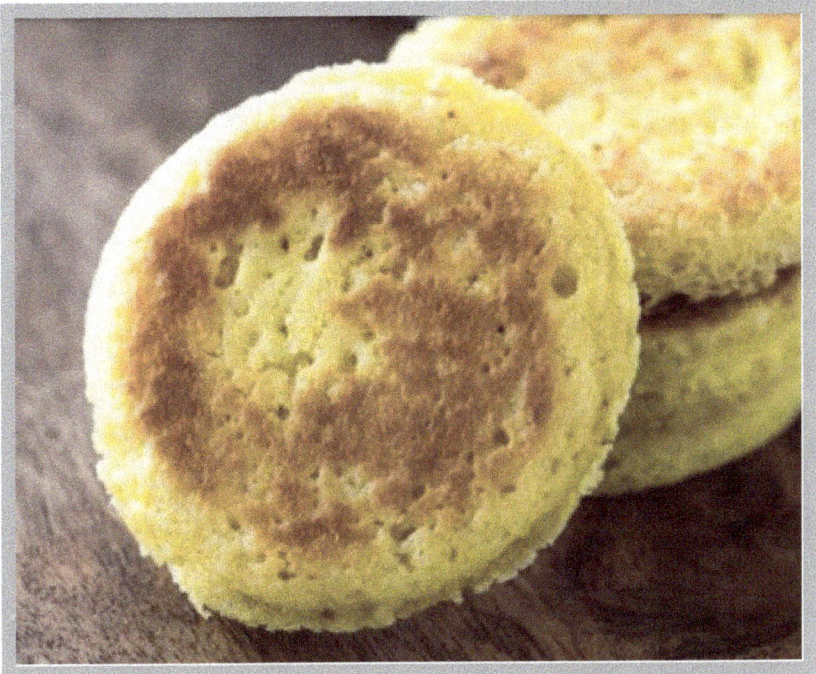

*P*reparation time: 1 min

Cooking time: 1 min

Ready in: 2 min

Ingredients:

1. 3 tablespoons or 1 tablespoon coconut flour

2. 1 tablespoon butter or oil

3. 1 medium/large egg

4. 1/2 teaspoon double-acting baking powder

Instructions:

1. At first, melt butter in a microwave-safe bowl or ramekin and add the almond flour, egg, and baking powder to the butter. Then beat with a fork until completely mix.

2. Do microwave for about 90 seconds, until firm. Then run a knife along the edge and flip over a plate to release. Do slice in half, then toast in the toaster or in a skillet.

3. for Bake: Pre-heat oven to 375F. Do Bake in a ramekin for 10-12 minutes or until cooked through.

18. KETO BREAD 4

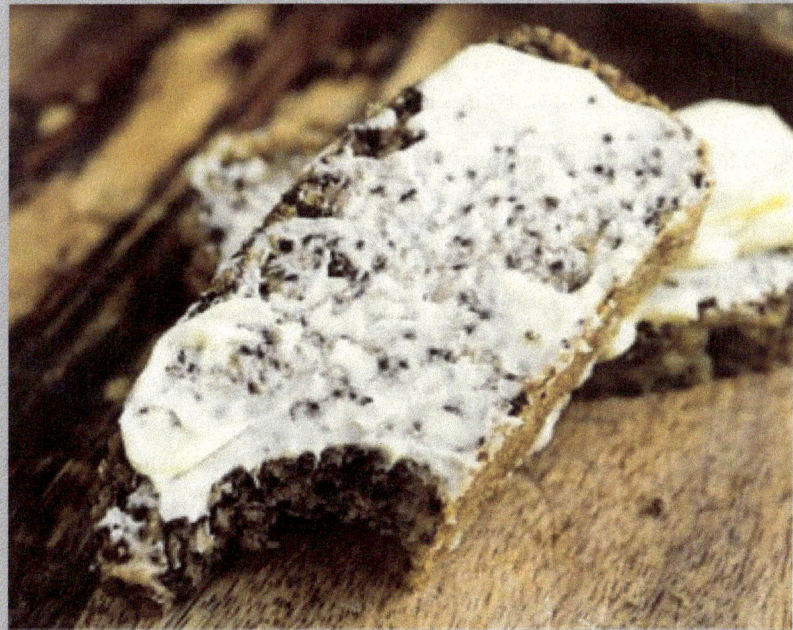

*P*reparation time: 5 min

Cooking time: 30 min

Ready in: 35 min

Ingredients:

1. 4 (4) Eggs

2. 1 cup (112 g) Superfine Almond Flour

3. 1/2 cup (85 g) Black Chia Seeds,

4. 1/4 cup (62.5 g) Unsweetened Almond Milk

5. 1/4 cup (54.5 g) Coconut Oil or Melted Butter

6. 2 teaspoons (2 teaspoons) Baking Soda

7. 1/2 teaspoon (0.5 teaspoons) Salt

Instructions:

1. At first, preheat the oven to 350F.

2. Then grease a 4-cup loaf pan (8 x 4 inch) and set aside. Please do not use a larger loaf pan as the bread will be very flat. Then you might choose to bake it in two mini pans if you want your bread to rise more.

3. Do mix all ingredients in a bowl and stir until the batter is well mixed and not lumpy.

4. Now pour into the greased loaf pan and bake for 28 minutes. Please allow the bread to rest in the pan for 10 minutes. Then remove and place on a rack to fully cool it.

5. If you just can't wait for it, get out some butter and have at it!

19. 90-SECOND KETO BREAD 2

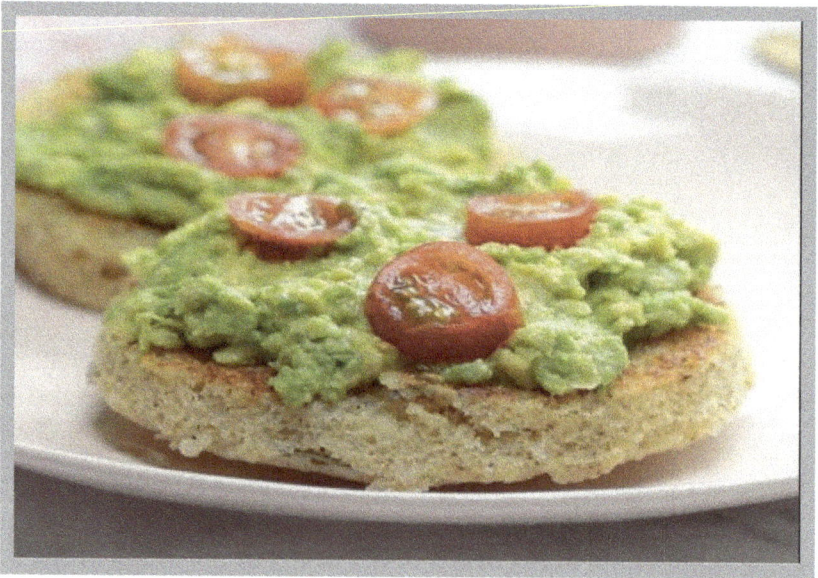

*P*reparation time: 2 min

Cooking time: 3 min

Ready in: 5 min

. . .

Ingredients:

1. 3 tablespoons almond flour

2. ½ teaspoon baking powder

3. ¼ cup shredded parmesan cheese (30 g)

4. 1 teaspoon fresh rosemary, chopped

5. ½ teaspoon garlic powder

6. Salt, to taste

7. Pepper, to taste

8. Unsalted butter, melted

9. 1 large egg, beaten

Instructions:

1. at first in a microwave-safe ramekin or small bowl and combine the almond flour, baking powder, Parmesan, rosemary, garlic powder, salt, pepper, melted butter, and egg. Now stir everything together with a fork until smooth.

2. Do microwave on high for 90 seconds, until the bread has risen.

3. Then lets the bread cool in the ramekin and then serve as desired.

4. Enjoy!

20. GLUTEN-FREE & KETO BREAD WITH YEAST

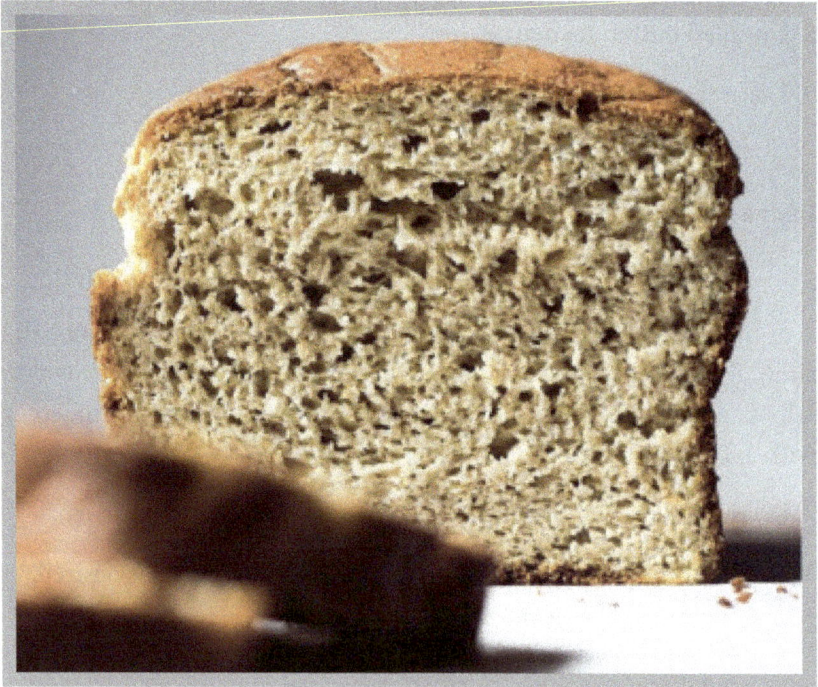

*P*reparation time: 15 min

Cooking time: 30 min

Ready in: 45 min

Ingredients:

1. 2 teaspoons active dry yeast

2. 2 teaspoons insulin or maple syrup, honey, to feed the yeast

3. 120 ml water lukewarm between 105-110°F

4. 168 g almond flour

5. 83 g golden flaxseed meal finely ground

6. 15 g whey protein isolate

7. 18 g husk finely ground

8. 2 teaspoons xanthan gum or 4 teaspoons ground flaxseed meal

9. 2 teaspoons baking powder

10. 1 teaspoon kosher salt

11. 1/4 teaspoon cream of tartar

12. 1/8 teaspoon ground ginger

13. 1 egg at room temperature

14. 110 g egg whites about 3, at room temperature

15. 56 g grass-fed unsalted butter or ghee, melted and cooled

16. 1 tablespoon apple cider vinegar

17. 58 g sour cream or coconut cream + 2 tsp apple cider vinegar

Instructions:

1. At first line, an 8.5 x 4.5-inch loaf pan with parchment paper (an absolute must!) and set aside.

2. Then add yeast and maple syrup (to feed the yeast, see notes) to a large bowl and heat up water to 105-110°F, and if you don't have a thermometer, it should only feel slightly warm to touch. Now pour water over yeast mixture, cover the bowl with a kitchen towel and allow resting for 5 minutes. Now the mixture should be bubbly if it doesn't start again (too cold water won't activate the yeast and too hot will kill it).

4. Do mix your flours while the yeast is proofing and add almond flour, flaxseed meal, whey protein powder, husk, xanthan gum, baking powder, salt, cream of tartar and ginger take a medium bowl and whisk until thoroughly mixed.

5. Then once your yeast is proofed, add in the egg, egg whites, lightly cooled melted butter, and vinegar. Do mix with an electric mixer for a couple of minutes until light and frothy. Then add the flour mixture in two batches, alternating with the sour cream and mixing until thoroughly incorporated. Now you want to mix thoroughly and quickly to activate the xanthan gum, though the dough will become thick as the flours absorb the moisture.

6. please transfer bread dough to prepared loaf pan, using a wet

spatula to even out the top and cover with a kitchen towel and place in a warm draft-free space for 50-60 minutes until the dough has risen just past the top of the loaf pan and keep in mind that if you use a larger loaf pan, it won't rise past the top.

7. Then preheat oven to 350°F/180°C while the dough is proofing, and if you're baking at high altitude, you'll want to bake it at 375°F/195°C.

8. Now place the loaf pan over a baking tray and transfer gently into the oven. Bake for 45-50 minutes until deep golden, covering with a loose foil dome at minute 15-20. Now just be sure that the foil isn't resting directly on the bread.

9. Do allow the bread to rest in the loaf pan for 5 minutes and transfer it to a cooling rack. Please don't sweat it!

10. Final stage: Keep stored in an airtight container (or tightly wrapped in cling film) at room temperature for 5-6 days, giving it a light toast before serving.

21. 90 SECOND KETO BREAD 3

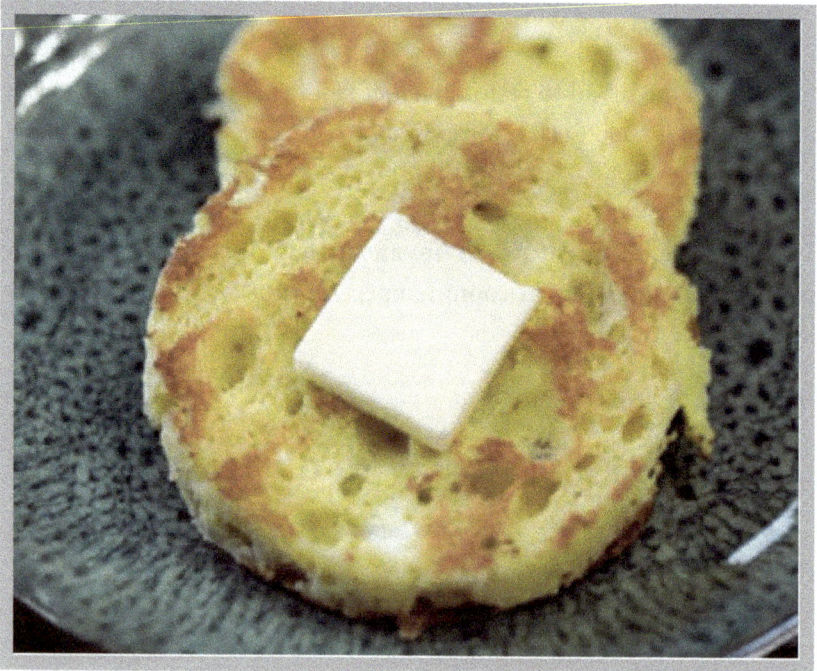

*P*reparation time: 1 min

Cooking time: 2 min

Ready in: 3 min

Ingredients:

1. 3 tablespoons almond flour

2. 1 egg

3. 1/2 teaspoon baking powder

4. 1/4 teaspoon salt

5. 1 tablespoon butter, melted

6. optional – 1 tablespoon butter

Instructions:

1. At first, pour all the ingredients in a microwave-safe bowl (Our container measures 4 inches wide at the bottom) use a fork or a small whisk to whisk it together in a small bowl.

2. Now place in the microwave for 90 seconds.

3. Then remove from microwave and allow cooling slightly.

4. Final part: Then cut in half.

22. THE BEST KETO BREAD RECIPE 2

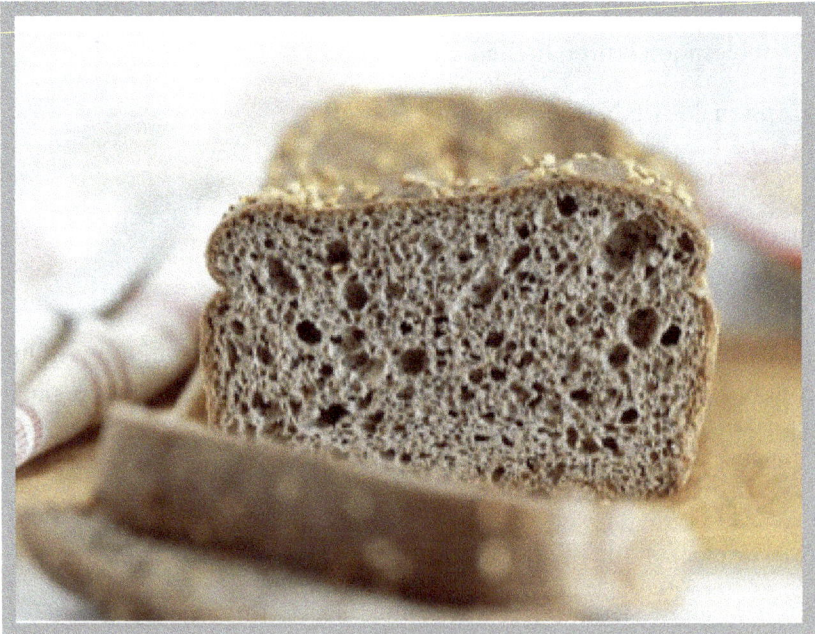

*P*reparation time: 10 min

Cooking time: 65 min

Ready in: 75 min

Ingredients

1. 1 1/4 cups (5oz/143g) almond flour

2. 5 tablespoons husk powder

3. 2 teaspoons baking powder

4. 1 teaspoon salt

5. 2 teaspoons apple cider vinegar

6. 1 cup (8floz/225ml) boiling water

7. 3 egg whites

8. 2 tablespoons sesame seeds, optional

Instructions:

1. Please Preheat your oven your oven to 350°F (180°C), then butter and line a 9x5 inch loaf tin with parchment paper.

2. Take a large bowl to combine the almond flour, husk, baking powder, and salt.

3. Then add the egg whites and apple cider vinegar to the dry ingredients with an electric mixer on medium speed until the paste-like dough is formed.

4. Now while mixing on low speed, stream in the boiling water. Do

turn the speed up to high and mix for about 30 seconds, or until the dough forms an elastic play-dough like mixture. Please be careful not to over-mix!

5. Now transfer the dough to the prepared baking tin and smooth the top and lastly, sprinkle over the sesame seeds.

6. Please bake the bread for 55-65 minutes or until the top has risen and puffed up like a traditional sandwich loaf.

7. Then remove the bread from the oven and allow cooling slightly before transferring to a cooling rack.

8. Final stage: Once cooled slice and enjoy! Please store the bread covered at room temperature for 2 days. Then after 2 days, I suggest storing it in the fridge for no longer than another 2 days.

23. BEST KETO BREAD RECIPE WITHOUT EGGS

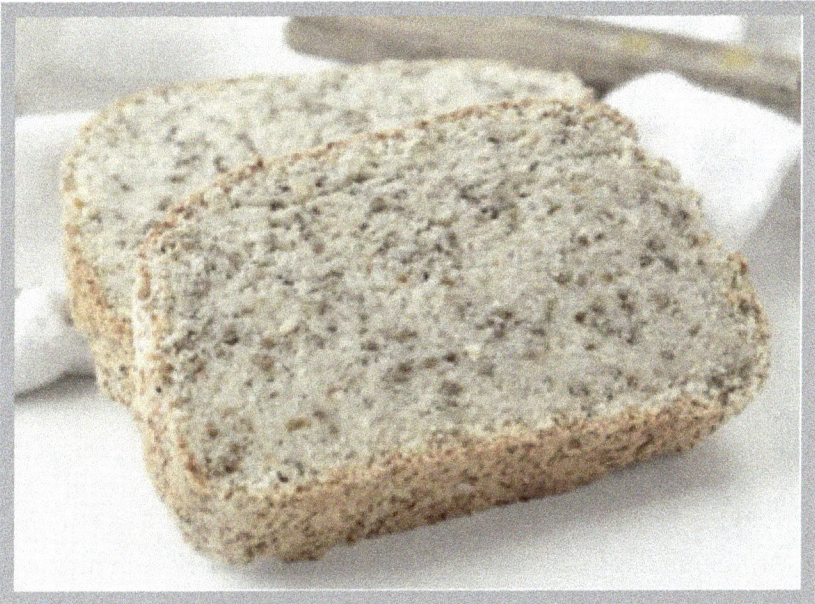

*P*reparation time: 15 min

Cooking time: 60 min

Ready in: 75 min

Ingredients:

Dry ingredients

1. 4.3 oz coconut flour packed, leveled (123g or 1 cup)

2. 2.1 oz almond flour (60g or 1/2 cup)

3. 0.95 oz husk (27 g or1/3cup)

4. 0.91 oz chia seeds (26 g or 2 tablespoons)

5. 1/2 teaspoon salt

Liquid ingredients

1. 18 fl.oz lukewarm water (530 ml or 2 1/4 cup)

2. 2 teaspoons apple cider vinegar (10 ml)

3. 2 teaspoon baking powder

Instructions:

1. At first, preheat oven 180C (350F), fan mode works the best and faster; otherwise, use conventional baking mode and line a loaf pan 9 inches x 5 inches with parchment paper.

2. Then measure all your ingredients carefully before you start, and I highly recommend weighing your ingredients in grams or oz for precision rather than cups.

3. Please use a large mixing bowl; whisk together all the dry ingredients.

4. Then add apple cider vinegar and lukewarm water.

5. Please combine with a spoon at first, and it will be very liquid and dry out as you go. After 40 seconds, the dough is moist, not liquid, and slightly crumbles apart. Then knead the dough, press/squeeze with your hands for at least 1.20 minutes, or until you are able to form a ball.

6. Then form a dough ball and set aside on the benchtop for 11 minutes to let the fiber absorb all the water and hold the ingredients together.

7. The dough should be soft, elastic, a slightly moist but hold perfectly together.

8. Now shape a cylinder, bread loaf shape. Please don't press too much the dough, it is gluten-free bread, it won't rise, and the shape you give will be the shape you get.

9. I give you another option is to shape 14 small buns to make bread rolls. If you so bake on a cookie sheet covered with parchment paper. Then it will bake faster only 35 minutes on the bottom rack

10. Now place the loaf onto the prepared loaf pan covered with parchment paper.

11. If it cracks appears on top, wet your fingers with water and massage top of the bread to fix cracks and sprinkle one tablespoon of sesame seeds or poppy seeds to decorate (optional)

. . .

12. do bake on the bottom rack of the oven (first rack from the bottom) for 45 minutes, then switch to the middle rack for 15 extra minutes, and you can add a piece of foil paper on top of the loaf if the color gets too brown.

13. Now insert a skewer in the middle of the bread to check the texture, and it should come out dry with no or few crumbs on it.

14. Final stage: Remove from the oven and cool on a rack for 4 hours or overnight before slicing.

24. KETO BREAD ROLLS

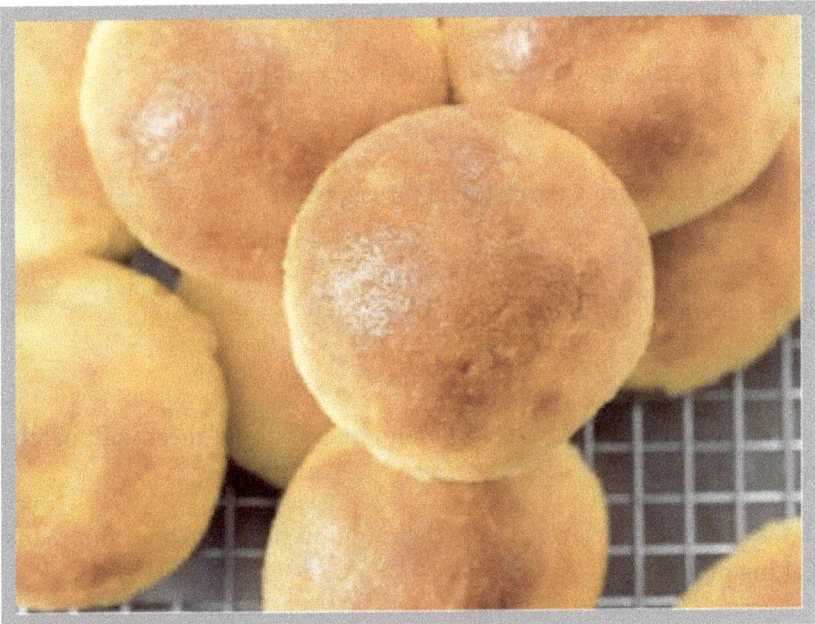

*P*reparation time: 15 min

Cooking time: 21 min

Ready in: 36 min

Ingredients:

1. 1 1/2 cups part-skim low moisture shredded mozzarella cheese

2. 2 oz full-fat cream cheese

3. 1 1/3 cups superfine almond flour

4. 2 tbsp coconut flour

5. 1 1/2 tbsp aluminum-free double-acting baking powder

6. 3 large eggs one egg is reserved for egg wash

Instructions:

1. Turn on preheat oven to 350°F and line a baking sheet with parchment paper.

2. take a small bowl, whisk together almond flour, coconut flour, and baking powder.

3. Then add mozzarella and cream cheese to a large microwave-safe bowl and cover the cream cheese with mozzarella. Now please melt in the microwave at 30-second intervals. After every 30 seconds, stir cheese until cheese is completely melted and uniform and resembles

dough in appearance. It should only take around one minute total cooking time. Please do not try to microwave the full time at once because some of the cheese will overcook, and you can also melt the cheeses over the stove in a double boiler.

4. Please allow cheese dough to cool slightly (only a few minutes) so that it is still warm to the touch but not too hot, and if the cheese is too hot, it will cook the eggs. Please remember to avoid letting the cheese cool down completely because then it will turn hard, and you will not be able to blend it with the other dough ingredients.

5. Now add cheese, 2 eggs, and almond flour mixture into a food processor with a dough blade attachment. Then pulse at high speed until the dough is uniform, and the dough will be quite sticky, which is normal?

6. Then scoop out dough with a spatula and place onto a large sheet of plastic wrap. Do cover the dough in plastic wrap and knead a few times with the dough inside the plastic wrap until you have a uniform dough ball. Now lightly coat your hands with oil and divide the dough into 8 equal parts. Do roll each dough between your palms until it forms a smooth round ball. Now place dough balls onto a baking sheet, spaced 2 inches apart.

7. Then add the final egg to a small bowl and whisk and generously brush the surface of rolls with egg wash.

8. Do bake rolls for about 21-23 minutes in the middle rack of your oven, or until rolls are golden brown. Remind one thing rolls are best eaten hot.

25. LOW CARB KETO BREAD

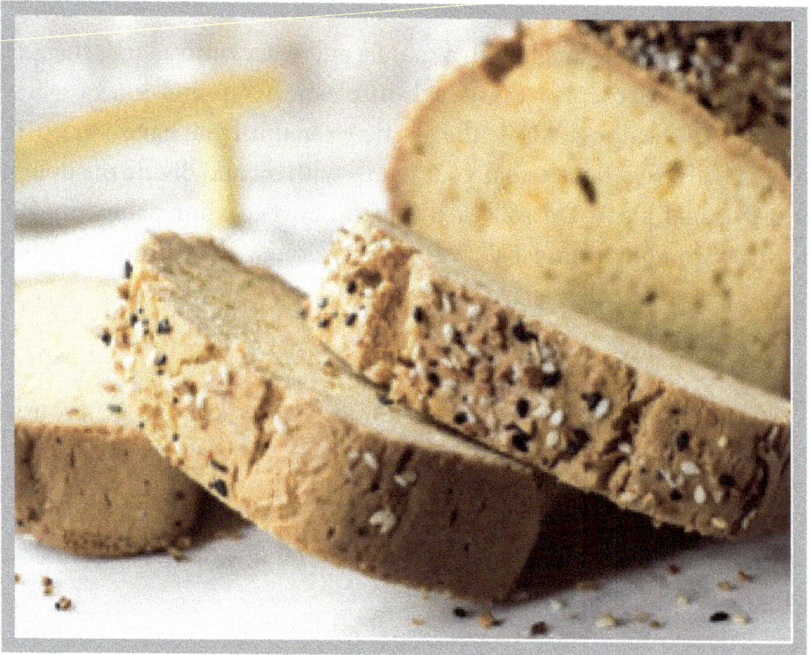

*P*reparation time: 5 min

Cooking time: 33 min

Ready in: 38 min

Ingredients:

1. 1 cup macadamia nuts unsalted & roasted

2. 5 good quality eggs

3. ½ teaspoon kosher salt

4. Zest of half a lemon

5. 1 teaspoon baking soda

6. 1 tablespoon lemon juice

7. 1 cup softened coconut butter

8. 1 teaspoon baking powder

9. 1-2 tablespoons everything bagel seasoning

Instructions:

1. First stage: preheat oven to 350F and make sure the oven rack is set in the middle of the oven.

2. Then add the macadamia nuts to a food processor or a powerful blender and process for about 32 seconds, until almost creamy.

. . .

3. Then while the machine is running, add the eggs one at a time, making sure each one has been incorporated into the batter before adding the next one.

4. Please turn the machine off and add the salt, lemon zest, baking soda, and lemon juice right on top of the baking soda to activate it. Do turn the machine on and process for another 20 seconds.

5. Then turn the machine off and add the softened coconut butter process until smooth and creamy.

6. Now turn the machine off and add the baking powder and process for 15-20 seconds and adding the baking powder will ensure that the bread doesn't turn greenish in color. It's very important to mix it at the end (not when you're adding the baking soda and lemon juice, as that will change the texture of your bread).

7. Then line the inside of a non-stick 10 x 4.5-inch bread or meatloaf tin with parchment paper. If you don't have parchment paper, then rub the inside with coconut oil or avocado oil or sprays it with a cooking spray. Please pour the batter into the tin and tap it on the counter a couple of times and sprinkle as much of the everything bagel seasoning as you would like. You can use your finger to press it down into the batter gently, so it does not fall off.

8. Do bake in the oven for 40-45 minutes, or until nicely golden brown on top. Now remove from oven, allow sitting in the tin for 5 minutes, and then lifting bread out using the parchment paper and transfer to a cooling rack for 10 minutes.

9. Final stage: slice the bread and enjoy!

26. 90 SECOND KETO BREAD 3

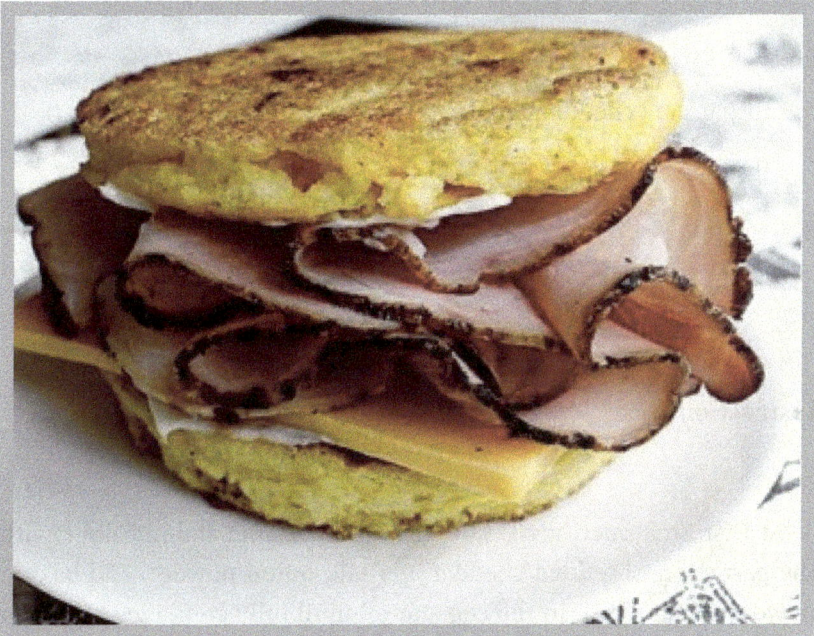

*P*reparation time: 2 min

Cooking time: 6 min

Ready in: 8 min

Ingredients:

1. 3 tbsp almond flour

2. 1 pinch onion powder

3. 1 pinch sea salt

4. 1/4 tsp baking powder

5. 1 tbsp grated parmesan cheese

6. 1 tbsp grated cheddar cheese

7. 1 tbsp olive oil

8. 1 egg

9. 1/2 tbsp butter

Instructions:

1. At first, in a microwave-safe dish, combine the almond flour with the parmesan, shredded cheddar, sea salt, onion powder, and baking powder. Then whisk in the egg and oil until fully combined and then microwave for 90 seconds and it will have puffed up in the microwave and look like a spongy egg creation!

2. Then heat butter in a skillet on medium-high. Please allow 'bread' to cool for 2 minutes, then cut in half, horizontally, to form two thinner bread slices. Do fry in a skillet until the bread is nice and toasty on both sides. Let's cool for a couple of minutes before using for burgers or sandwiches.

27. THE BEST KETO CLOUD BREAD RECIPE

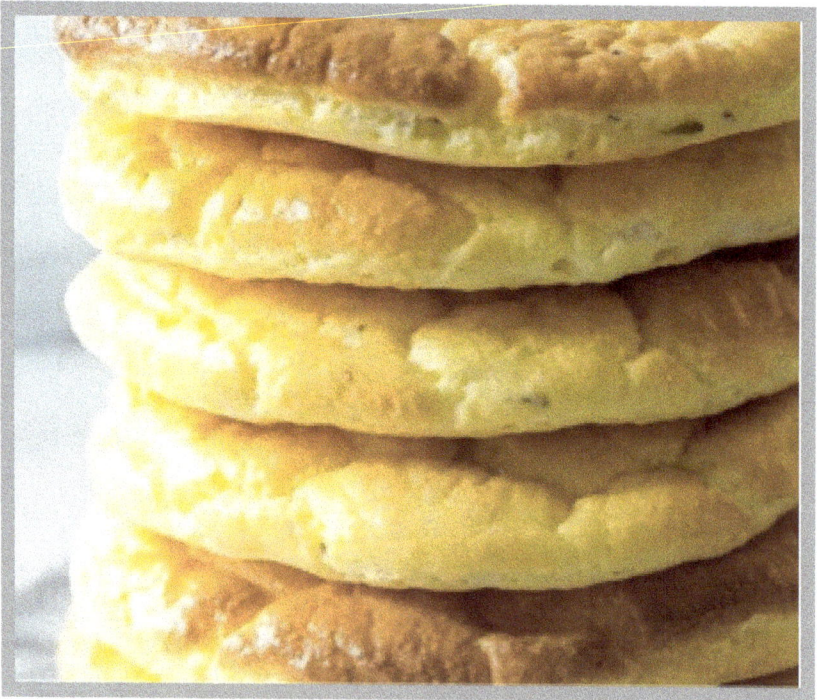

*P*reparation time: 10 min

Cooking time: 15 min

Ready in: 25 min

Ingredients:

1. 4 large eggs, separated

2. 1/2 teaspoon cream of tartar

3. 2 ounces low-fat cream cheese

4. 1 teaspoon Italian herb seasoning

5. 1/2 teaspoon sea salt

6. 1/4 - 1/2 teaspoon garlic powder

Instructions:

1. At first, preheat the oven to 300 degrees F, and if you have a convection oven, set on the convict. Then you have to line two large baking sheets with parchment paper.

2. Then separate the egg whites and egg yolks and place the whites in a stand mixer with a whip attachment. And add the cream of tartar and beat on high until the froth turns into firm meringue peaks. Please move to a separate bowl.

3. Then place the cream cheese in the empty stand mixing bowl and beat on high to soften. Then please add the egg yolks one at a time to incorporate and scrape the bowl and beat until the mixture is

completely smooth. Then beat in the seasoning, salt, and garlic powder.

4. Then gently fold the firm meringue into the yolk mixture and Try to deflate the meringue as little as possible, so the mixture is still firm and foamy. Now spoon 1/4 cup portions of the foam onto the baking sheets and spread into even 4-inch circles, 3/4 inch high. Please make sure to leave space around each circle.

5. Do bake on convict for 15-20 minutes or in a conventional oven for up to 30 minutes, and the bread should be golden on the outside and firm. Let's cool for several minutes on the baking sheets, then move and serve!

28. EASY KETO SANDWICH BREAD RECIPE

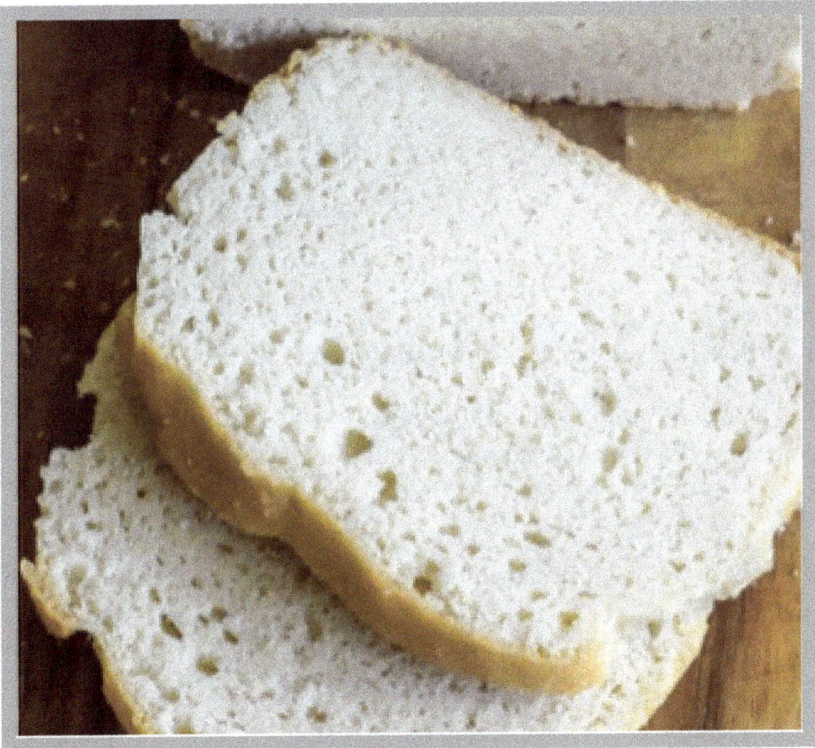

*P*reparation time: 5 min

Cooking time: 25 min

Ready in: 30 min

Ingredients:

1. 2 1/2 cups almond flour

2. 2 cups whey protein

3. 1 tbsp gum

4. 3 tsp baking powder

5. 1/2 tsp salt

6. 1 1/4 cups warm water

Instructions:

1. At first, in a large mixing bowl, stir together the dry ingredients.

2. Then slowly add in the water and stir with a wooden spoon, stirring slowly as you add water until your dough comes together.

3. Now pour bread dough into a loaf pan that has been lined with parchment paper or greased well (be sure to check your cooking spray to ensure it is, in fact, gluten-free.)

4. Do bake at 375°F for 20 to 25 minutes - until puffy and golden

brown. Now you will see air bubbles on the sides of the bread, similar to the way the bread looks inside.

5. Then remove from oven and let cool completely on a rack before slicing.

6. Final stage: only slice off the bread you're going to eat - pre-slicing bread will cause it to dry out or mold faster.

7. Enjoy.

29. KETO COCONUT-FLOUR BREAD

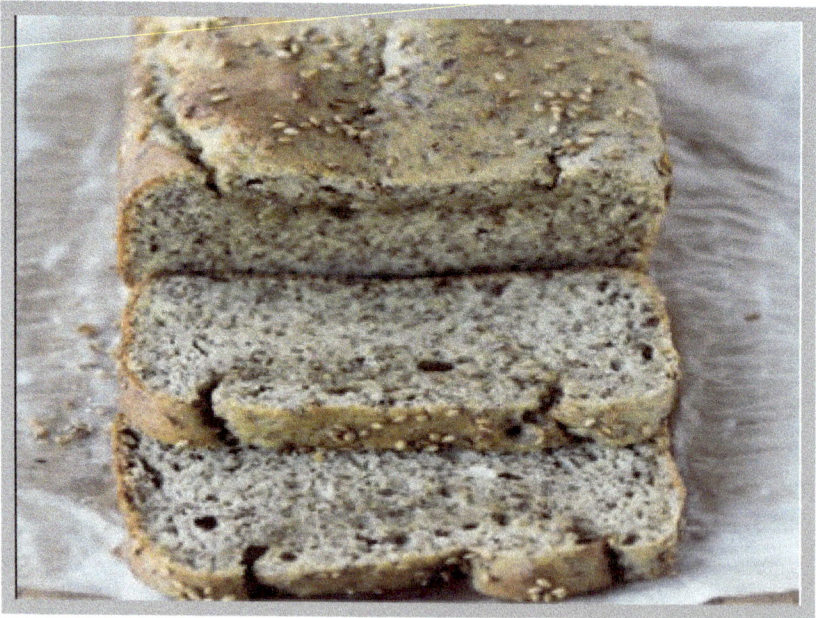

$\mathcal{P}$reparation time: 5 min

Cooking time: 25 min

Ready in: 30 min

Ingredients:

1. ½ cup coconut flour

2. ¼ tsp sea salt

3. ¼ tsp baking powder

4. 6 eggs

5. ½ cups melted coconut oil

Instructions:

1. Please preheat the oven to 350°F (175°C).
2. Take a medium-sized bowl, sift together the dry ingredients.
3. Now slowly add the wet ingredients into the dry ingredients and stir until very smooth.
4. Then grease a small bread pan and fill about ⅔ of the way full with batter. Do bake for 40-50 minutes, or until a toothpick comes out clean.

30. KETO BREAD: A LOW-CARB BREAD RECIPE

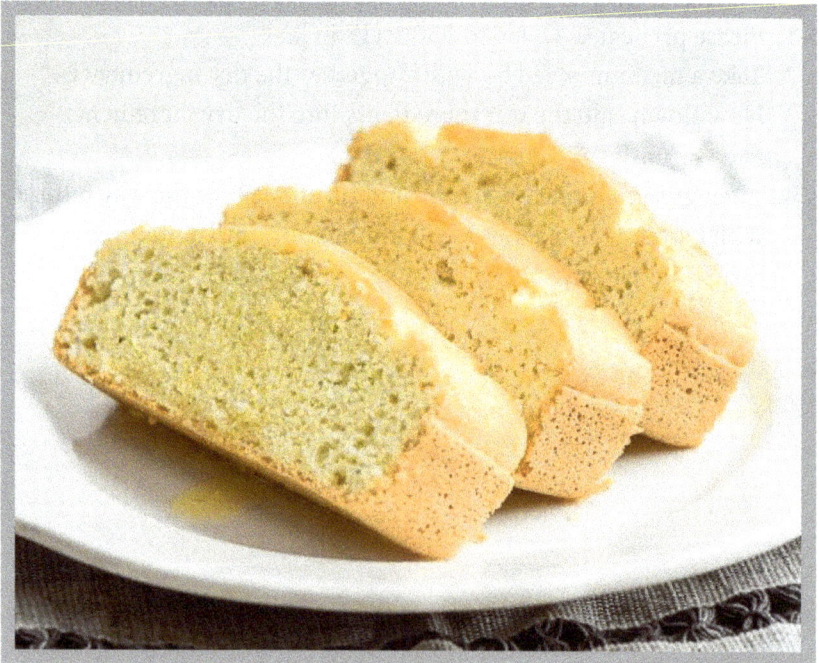

*P*reparation time: 10 min

Cooking time: 30 min

Ready in: 40 min

Ingredients:

1. 1½ cups almond flour

2. 6 egg whites

3. ¼ teaspoon cream of tartar

4. 3–4 tablespoons butter, melted

5. ¾ teaspoon baking soda

6. 3 teaspoons apple cider vinegar

7. 2 tablespoons coconut flour

Instructions:

1. Please preheat the oven to 375 F.

2. Then add the cream of tartar to the egg white mixture and, using a hand mixer, whip the eggs until soft peaks are formed.

3. Now add the almond flour, butter, baking soda, apple cider vinegar, and coconut flour to a food processor, blending until well-incorporated.

4. Do place the mix into a bowl and gently fold in the egg white

mixture.

5. And then, Grease an 8x4 loaf pan and pour in the bread mixture.

6. Do bake for 30 minutes.

7. Enjoy!!!!